SIMPLEST TYPE 2 DIABETES COOKBOOK FOR BEGINNERS

Easy & Delicious Recipes for Everyday Life

T. John

COPYRIGHT PAGE

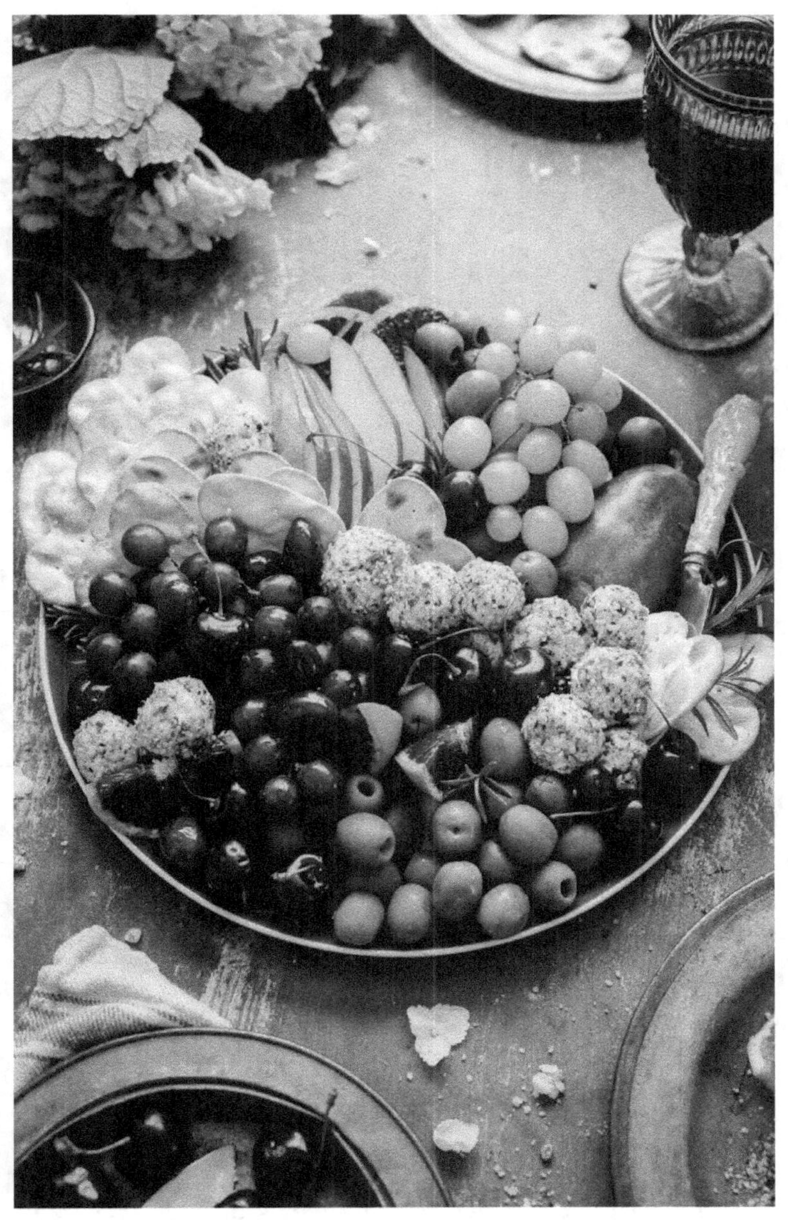

TABLE OF CONTENTS

INTRODUCTION

Imagine a boat bobbing on a sugar-sweet sea. The sun beats down, the waves lap lazily, and life seems pretty good. But below the surface lurks a storm—a brewing imbalance in the body's ability to handle this very sweetness. This, my friend, is the ocean of Type 2 Diabetes.

Now, you're not alone in this boat. Millions navigate these sugary waters, and while it may seem daunting, remember, a trusty seafaring tool—a healthy diet—can help chart a course to calmer waters. But before we raise the sails, let's understand the storm we face.

Type 2 Diabetes, unlike its pirate-like cousin Type 1, isn't about an insulin shortage. It's about resistance. Think of insulin as the captain, steering glucose (sugar) from your food into your cells, for energy. In Type 2, the crew—your cells—have become rebellious, ignoring the captain's orders. Glucose builds up, creating that ocean swell, threatening to swamp your health.

So, what's a diabetic sailor to do? Grab that healthy diet harpoon and reel in some key changes:

- **Swap out refined carbs for whole grains**: Ditch the white bread and sugary cereals. Think whole-wheat, brown rice, quinoa – these complex carbs release glucose slowly, keeping the waves gentle.
- **Befriend the veggie patch**: Load up on leafy greens, colorful peppers, and juicy tomatoes. These nutrient-packed pirates fight free radicals and keep your ship shipshape.
- **Make friends with lean protein**: Chicken, fish, beans – these hearty mates provide sustained energy without spiking your blood sugar.
- **Limit the sugary sirens**: Candy, cakes, sodas – these sugary temptresses sing a false song of pleasure. Steer clear, or your blood sugar will hit the rocks!
- **Portion control is your compass**: Don't overload your galley. Smaller, more frequent meals keep the glucose current calm and steady.
- **Hydration is your anchor**: Water is the ocean's lifeblood, and yours too. Keep that canteen full to

flush out excess sugar and keep your system humming.

Remember, this journey isn't a solo sprint. Seek guidance from your doctor and a registered dietitian, your fellow seafarers. They'll help tailor your diet to your specific needs and keep you on course.

Finally, don't forget the beauty of this journey. Savor the sweetness of a ripe mango, the earthy comfort of lentils, the laughter shared over a healthy meal. Celebrate the small victories, the calmer days, the newfound strength you discover within. With a healthy diet as your compass, you'll navigate the sweet sea of Type 2 Diabetes with grace and resilience, finding calm waters and a life richly lived.

So, raise your fork, my friend, and set sail toward a healthier horizon. The ocean may be sweet, but the journey with a healthy diet is one worth taking.

Chapter 1: 30 Day Meal Plan

Week 1:

Day 1:

- Breakfast: Nutrient-Packed Oatmeal Bowl
- Lunch: Grilled Chicken Salad with Lemon Vinaigrette
- Dinner: Baked Salmon with Dill Sauce
- Snacks: Guacamole with Veggie Sticks
- Dessert: Berry and Greek Yogurt Popsicles

Day 2:

- Breakfast: Veggie and Cheese Omelette
- Lunch: Quinoa and Black Bean Bowl
- Dinner: Spaghetti Squash with Turkey Bolognese
- Snacks: Greek Yogurt and Berry Parfait
- Dessert: Dark Chocolate-Dipped Strawberries

Day 3:

- Breakfast: Greek Yogurt Parfait with Berries
- Lunch: Turkey and Veggie Wrap

- Dinner: Lemon Herb Grilled Chicken

- Snacks: Hummus and Whole Wheat Pita

- Dessert: Baked Apples with Cinnamon

Day 4:

- Breakfast: Whole Wheat Pancakes with Sugar-Free Syrup

- Lunch: Lentil Soup with Spinach

- Dinner: Eggplant and Tomato Stacks

- Snacks: Cucumber and Tuna Bites

- Dessert: Sugar-Free Mango Sorbet

Day 5:

- Breakfast: Avocado Toast with Poached Egg

- Lunch: Shrimp and Vegetable Stir-Fry

- Dinner: Blackened Tilapia with Mango Salsa

- Snacks: Edamame with Sea Salt

- Dessert: Almond Flour Chocolate Chip Cookies

Day 6:

- Breakfast: Chia Seed Pudding with Almonds

- Lunch: Chickpea and Avocado Salad

- Dinner: Stuffed Bell Peppers with Quinoa

- Snacks: Almond and Cranberry Trail Mix

- Dessert: Chia Seed Chocolate Pudding

Day 7:

- Breakfast: Quinoa Breakfast Bowl

- Lunch: Turkey and Sweet Potato Chili

- Dinner: Teriyaki Tofu Stir-Fry

- Snacks: Caprese Skewers with Cherry Tomatoes

- Dessert: Grilled Peaches with Honey

Week 2:

Day 8:

- Breakfast: Spinach and Feta Breakfast Wrap

- Lunch: Caprese Salad with Balsamic Glaze

- Dinner: Cilantro Lime Shrimp Skewers

- Snacks: Apple Slices with Peanut Butter

- Dessert: Vanilla Chia Seed Pudding

Day 9:

- Breakfast: Cottage Cheese and Fruit Bowl

- Lunch: Broccoli and Brown Rice Casserole

- Dinner: Sweet Potato and Chickpea Curry
- Snacks: Cottage Cheese and Pineapple Cups
- Dessert: Lemon Blueberry Muffins (Low-Sugar)

Day 10:

- Breakfast: Sweet Potato Hash with Turkey Sausage
- Lunch: Tofu and Vegetable Skewers
- Dinner: Grilled Portobello Mushrooms with Garlic
- Snacks: Roasted Red Pepper and Feta Dip
- Dessert: Avocado Chocolate Mousse

Day 11:

- Breakfast: Smoothie Bowl with Mixed Berries
- Lunch: Mediterranean Quinoa Salad
- Dinner: Turkey and Vegetable Casserole
- Snacks: Hard-Boiled Egg with Mustard
- Dessert: Pumpkin Spice Energy Bites

Day 12:

- Breakfast: Breakfast Burrito with Black Beans
- Lunch: Zucchini Noodles with Pesto
- Dinner: Lemon Garlic Butter Shrimp

- Snacks: Avocado and Tomato Salsa
- Dessert: Mixed Berry Crisp

Day 13:

- Breakfast: Almond Butter and Banana Sandwich
- Lunch: Chicken and Vegetable Lettuce Wraps
- Dinner: Ratatouille with Herbed Quinoa
- Snacks: Spinach and Artichoke Dip
- Dessert: Coconut Milk Rice Pudding

Day 14:

- Breakfast: Egg and Vegetable Muffins
- Lunch: Cauliflower Fried Rice
- Dinner: Baked Chicken Breast with Rosemary
- Snacks: Mixed Nuts and Seeds
- Dessert: Raspberry Almond Tarts

Week 3:

Day 15:

- Breakfast: Salmon and Avocado Bagel
- Lunch: Greek Chicken Souvlaki
- Dinner: Mexican Cauliflower Rice Bowl

- Snacks: Stuffed Mini Bell Peppers
- Dessert: Banana Walnut Muffins (No Added Sugar)

Day 16:

- Breakfast: Nutrient-Packed Oatmeal Bowl
- Lunch: Grilled Chicken Salad with Lemon Vinaigrette
- Dinner: Baked Salmon with Dill Sauce
- Snacks: Guacamole with Veggie Sticks
- Dessert: Berry and Greek Yogurt Popsicles

Day 17:

- Breakfast: Veggie and Cheese Omelette
- Lunch: Quinoa and Black Bean Bowl
- Dinner: Spaghetti Squash with Turkey Bolognese
- Snacks: Greek Yogurt and Berry Parfait
- Dessert: Dark Chocolate-Dipped Strawberries

Day 18:

- Breakfast: Greek Yogurt Parfait with Berries
- Lunch: Turkey and Veggie Wrap
- Dinner: Lemon Herb Grilled Chicken

- Snacks: Hummus and Whole Wheat Pita
- Dessert: Baked Apples with Cinnamon

Day 19:

- Breakfast: Whole Wheat Pancakes with Sugar-Free Syrup
- Lunch: Lentil Soup with Spinach
- Dinner: Eggplant and Tomato Stacks
- Snacks: Cucumber and Tuna Bites
- Dessert: Sugar-Free Mango Sorbet

Day 20:

- Breakfast: Avocado Toast with Poached Egg
- Lunch: Shrimp and Vegetable Stir-Fry
- Dinner: Blackened Tilapia with Mango Salsa
- Snacks: Edamame with Sea Salt
- Dessert: Almond Flour Chocolate Chip Cookies

Day 21:

- Breakfast: Chia Seed Pudding with Almonds
- Lunch: Chickpea and Avocado Salad
- Dinner: Stuffed Bell Peppers with Quinoa

- Snacks: Almond and Cranberry Trail Mix
- Dessert: Chia Seed Chocolate Pudding

Week 4:

Day 22:

- Breakfast: Quinoa Breakfast Bowl
- Lunch: Turkey and Sweet Potato Chili
- Dinner: Teriyaki Tofu Stir-Fry
- Snacks: Caprese Skewers with Cherry Tomatoes
- Dessert: Grilled Peaches with Honey

Day 23:

- Breakfast: Spinach and Feta Breakfast Wrap
- Lunch: Caprese Salad with Balsamic Glaze
- Dinner: Cilantro Lime Shrimp Skewers
- Snacks: Apple Slices with Peanut Butter
- Dessert: Vanilla Chia Seed Pudding

Day 24:

- Breakfast: Cottage Cheese and Fruit Bowl
- Lunch: Broccoli and Brown Rice Casserole
- Dinner: Sweet Potato and Chickpea Curry

- Snacks: Cottage Cheese and Pineapple Cups
- Dessert: Lemon Blueberry Muffins (Low-Sugar)

Day 25:

- Breakfast: Sweet Potato Hash with Turkey Sausage
- Lunch: Tofu and Vegetable Skewers
- Dinner: Grilled Portobello Mushrooms with Garlic
- Snacks: Roasted Red Pepper and Feta Dip
- Dessert: Avocado Chocolate Mousse

Day 26:

- Breakfast: Smoothie Bowl with Mixed Berries
- Lunch: Mediterranean Quinoa Salad
- Dinner: Turkey and Vegetable Casserole
- Snacks: Hard-Boiled Egg with Mustard
- Dessert: Pumpkin Spice Energy Bites

Day 27:

- Breakfast: Breakfast Burrito with Black Beans
- Lunch: Zucchini Noodles with Pesto
- Dinner: Lemon Garlic Butter Shrimp
- Snacks: Avocado and Tomato Salsa

- Dessert: Mixed Berry Crisp

Day 28:

- Breakfast: Almond Butter and Banana Sandwich
- Lunch: Chicken and Vegetable Lettuce Wraps
- Dinner: Ratatouille with Herbed Quinoa
- Snacks: Spinach and Artichoke Dip
- Dessert: Coconut Milk Rice Pudding

Day 29:

- Breakfast: Egg and Vegetable Muffins
- Lunch: Cauliflower Fried Rice
- Dinner: Baked Chicken Breast with Rosemary
- Snacks: Mixed Nuts and Seeds
- Dessert: Raspberry Almond Tarts

Day 30:

- Breakfast: Salmon and Avocado Bagel
- Lunch: Greek Chicken Souvlaki
- Dinner: Mexican Cauliflower Rice Bowl
- Snacks: Stuffed Mini Bell Peppers
- Dessert: Banana Walnut Muffins (No Added Sugar)

Chapter 2: Breakfast Recipes

In this chapter, we present breakfast recipes designed to kickstart your day with flavors that align with diabetes-friendly dietary needs.

Nutrient-Packed Oatmeal Bowl

Ingredients:

- 1/2 cup rolled oats
- 1 cup almond milk
- 1 tablespoon chia seeds
- 1/4 cup diced strawberries
- 1 tablespoon chopped nuts (walnuts or almonds)

Instructions:

1. In a saucepan, combine rolled oats and almond milk.
2. Bring to a simmer, stirring occasionally until oats are cooked.
3. Remove from heat, add chia seeds, and let it sit for 5 minutes.

4. Top with strawberries and nuts. Enjoy your hearty oatmeal bowl!

Nutrition Information:

- Calories: 300
- Protein: 10g
- Carbohydrates: 40g
- Fat: 12g
- Fiber: 8g
- Sugar: 5g
- Portion Size: 1 serving

Veggie and Cheese Omelette

Ingredients:

- 2 eggs
- 1/4 cup diced bell peppers
- 1/4 cup diced tomatoes
- 1/4 cup spinach leaves
- 1/4 cup shredded low-fat cheese

Instructions:

1. Whisk eggs in a bowl and pour into a preheated non-stick pan.
2. Add bell peppers, tomatoes, and spinach.
3. Sprinkle shredded cheese over the top and fold the omelette.
4. Cook until eggs are set. Serve your nutritious veggie and cheese omelette.

Nutrition Information:

- Calories: 220
- Protein: 15g
- Carbohydrates: 8g
- Fat: 14g
- Fiber: 2g
- Sugar: 3g
- Portion Size: 1 serving

Greek Yogurt Parfait with Berries

Ingredients:

- 1/2 cup Greek yogurt
- 1/4 cup granola (sugar-free)

- 1/4 cup mixed berries (blueberries, strawberries, raspberries)

Instructions:

1. In a glass, layer Greek yogurt, granola, and mixed berries.
2. Repeat the layers. Finish with a sprinkle of granola and berries on top.
3. Delight in the perfect harmony of flavors in your Greek yogurt parfait.

Nutrition Information:

- Calories: 250
- Protein: 15g
- Carbohydrates: 30g
- Fat: 8g
- Fiber: 4g
- Sugar: 12g
- Portion Size: 1 serving

Whole Wheat Pancakes with Sugar-Free Syrup

Ingredients:

- 1/2 cup whole wheat flour
- 1/2 cup almond milk
- 1 egg
- 1 teaspoon baking powder
- Sugar-free syrup for topping

Instructions:

1. Mix whole wheat flour, almond milk, egg, and baking powder in a bowl.
2. Pour batter onto a hot griddle to form pancakes.
3. Cook until bubbles form, then flip and cook the other side.
4. Top with sugar-free syrup. Savor your guilt-free whole wheat pancakes.

Nutrition Information:

- Calories: 280
- Protein: 10g
- Carbohydrates: 35g

- Fat: 8g
- Fiber: 5g
- Sugar: 2g
- Portion Size: 2 pancakes

Avocado Toast with Poached Egg

Ingredients:

- 1 slice whole grain bread
- 1/2 ripe avocado
- 1 poached egg
- Salt and pepper to taste

Instructions:

1. Toast the bread and spread mashed avocado on top.
2. Place a poached egg on the avocado.
3. Season with salt and pepper. Indulge in the creamy goodness of avocado toast.

Nutrition Information:

- Calories: 220
- Protein: 10g
- Carbohydrates: 15g

- Fat: 15g
- Fiber: 7g
- Sugar: 1g
- Portion Size: 1 serving

Chia Seed Pudding with Almonds

Ingredients:

- 3 tablespoons chia seeds
- 1 cup unsweetened almond milk
- 1/2 teaspoon vanilla extract
- 1 tablespoon sliced almonds
- Berries for topping

Instructions:

1. Mix chia seeds, almond milk, and vanilla extract in a jar.
2. Refrigerate for at least 4 hours or overnight.
3. Top with sliced almonds and berries. Enjoy the delightful chia seed pudding.

Nutrition Information:

- Calories: 180

- Protein: 5g

- Carbohydrates: 15g

- Fat: 10g

- Fiber: 8g

- Sugar: 2g

- Portion Size: 1 serving

Quinoa Breakfast Bowl

Ingredients:

- 1/2 cup cooked quinoa

- 1/4 cup unsweetened almond milk

- 1 tablespoon honey

- 1/4 cup sliced bananas

- 1 tablespoon chopped nuts (walnuts or almonds)

Instructions:

1. Combine cooked quinoa with almond milk and honey.

2. Top with sliced bananas and chopped nuts.

3. Drizzle with an extra touch of honey. Relish the wholesome quinoa breakfast bowl.

Nutrition Information:

- Calories: 280
- Protein: 7g
- Carbohydrates: 45g
- Fat: 8g
- Fiber: 5g
- Sugar: 15g
- Portion Size: 1 serving

Spinach and Feta Breakfast Wrap

Ingredients:

- 1 whole grain tortilla
- 2 eggs, scrambled
- Handful of fresh spinach
- 2 tablespoons crumbled feta cheese
- Salt and pepper to taste

Instructions:

1. Fill a tortilla with scrambled eggs, fresh spinach, and feta.
2. Season with salt and pepper.

3. Wrap it up and enjoy a savory spinach and feta breakfast delight.

Nutrition Information:

- Calories: 320
- Protein: 15g
- Carbohydrates: 25g
- Fat: 18g
- Fiber: 5g
- Sugar: 2g
- Portion Size: 1 wrap

Cottage Cheese and Fruit Bowl

Ingredients:

- 1/2 cup low-fat cottage cheese
- 1/2 cup mixed berries (strawberries, blueberries, raspberries)
- 1 tablespoon honey
- 1 tablespoon chopped nuts (almonds or walnuts)

Instructions:

1. Combine cottage cheese and mixed berries in a bowl.

2. Drizzle with honey and sprinkle chopped nuts on top.

3. Enjoy a protein-packed cottage cheese and fruit bowl.

Nutrition Information:

- Calories: 220
- Protein: 15g
- Carbohydrates: 25g
- Fat: 8g
- Fiber: 4g
- Sugar: 18g
- Portion Size: 1 serving

Sweet Potato Hash with Turkey Sausage

Ingredients:

- 1 cup sweet potatoes, diced
- 1/2 cup lean turkey sausage, crumbled
- 1/4 cup red bell pepper, diced
- 1/4 cup onion, chopped
- 1 tablespoon olive oil

- Salt and pepper to taste

Instructions:

1. In a skillet, heat olive oil and sauté sweet potatoes until golden.

2. Add turkey sausage, bell pepper, and onion. Cook until vegetables are tender.

3. Season with salt and pepper. Savor the flavorful sweet potato hash.

Nutrition Information:

- Calories: 280
- Protein: 12g
- Carbohydrates: 25g
- Fat: 15g
- Fiber: 5g
- Sugar: 6g
- Portion Size: 1 serving

Smoothie Bowl with Mixed Berries

Ingredients:

- 1/2 cup mixed berries (strawberries, blueberries, raspberries)
- 1/2 banana, frozen
- 1/2 cup Greek yogurt
- 1/4 cup almond milk
- Toppings: granola, sliced almonds, chia seeds

Instructions:

1. Blend mixed berries, frozen banana, Greek yogurt, and almond milk until smooth.
2. Pour into a bowl and top with granola, sliced almonds, and chia seeds.
3. Dive into the refreshing goodness of a mixed berry smoothie bowl.

Nutrition Information:

- Calories: 250
- Protein: 15g
- Carbohydrates: 35g
- Fat: 8g

- Fiber: 8g

- Sugar: 15g

- Portion Size: 1 serving

Breakfast Burrito with Black Beans

Ingredients:

- 1 whole grain tortilla

- 1/2 cup black beans, cooked

- 2 eggs, scrambled

- 1/4 cup salsa

- 2 tablespoons shredded low-fat cheese

Instructions:

1. Fill a tortilla with black beans, scrambled eggs, salsa, and shredded cheese.

2. Wrap it up and warm in a skillet until cheese is melted.

3. Enjoy a satisfying and protein-rich breakfast burrito.

Nutrition Information:

- Calories: 320

- Protein: 20g

- Carbohydrates: 30g

- Fat: 14g

- Fiber: 8g

- Sugar: 3g

- Portion Size: 1 burrito

Almond Butter and Banana Sandwich

Ingredients:

- 2 slices whole grain bread

- 2 tablespoons almond butter

- 1 banana, sliced

- 1 teaspoon honey (optional)

Instructions:

1. Spread almond butter on one side of each bread slice.

2. Arrange banana slices on one slice and drizzle with honey if desired.

3. Top with the second slice to make a delicious almond butter and banana sandwich.

Nutrition Information:

- Calories: 320
- Protein: 8g
- Carbohydrates: 45g
- Fat: 15g
- Fiber: 8g
- Sugar: 15g
- Portion Size: 1 sandwich

Egg and Vegetable Muffins

Ingredients:

- 4 eggs
- 1/2 cup mixed vegetables (bell peppers, spinach, tomatoes)
- 1/4 cup feta cheese, crumbled
- Salt and pepper to taste

Instructions:

1. Preheat the oven to 350°F (175°C). Grease a muffin tin.
2. In a bowl, beat eggs and mix in vegetables and feta cheese.

3. Pour the mixture into muffin cups and bake for 15-20 minutes until set.

4. Season with salt and pepper. Enjoy these portable egg and vegetable muffins.

Nutrition Information:

- Calories: 180
- Protein: 12g
- Carbohydrates: 5g
- Fat: 12g
- Fiber: 2g
- Sugar: 2g
- Portion Size: 2 muffins

Salmon and Avocado Bagel

Ingredients:

- 1 whole grain bagel, sliced and toasted
- 3 ounces smoked salmon
- 1/2 avocado, sliced
- 1 tablespoon cream cheese (optional)

Instructions:

1. Spread cream cheese on toasted bagel slices if desired.
2. Top with smoked salmon and avocado slices.
3. Revel in the delightful flavors of a salmon and avocado bagel.

Nutrition Information:

- Calories: 320
- Protein: 20g
- Carbohydrates: 30g
- Fat: 15g
- Fiber: 8g
- Sugar: 2g
- Portion Size: 1 bagel

This chapter is crafted with lunch recipes that are not only delicious but also considerate of dietary needs. Each recipe is designed to provide balanced nutrition while keeping the flavors enticing.

Grilled Chicken Salad with Lemon Vinaigrette

Ingredients:

- 2 boneless, skinless chicken breasts
- 4 cups mixed salad greens
- 1 cup cherry tomatoes, halved
- 1 cucumber, sliced
- 1/4 cup red onion, thinly sliced
- 2 tablespoons feta cheese, crumbled

Instructions:

1. Grill chicken breasts until cooked thoroughly.
2. Slice grilled chicken into strips.

3. In a large bowl, combine salad greens, cherry tomatoes, cucumber, red onion, and grilled chicken.

4. Drizzle with lemon vinaigrette and toss gently.

5. Top with crumbled feta cheese.

Nutrition Information (per serving):

- Calories: 350

- Protein: 30g

- Carbohydrates: 15g

- Fat: 18g

- Fiber: 5g

- Sugar: 5g

- Portion Size: 1 serving

Quinoa and Black Bean Bowl

Ingredients:

- 1 cup quinoa, cooked

- 1 can black beans, drained and rinsed

- 1 cup corn kernels

- 1 avocado, diced

- 1/4 cup fresh cilantro, chopped

Instructions:

1. In a bowl, combine cooked quinoa, black beans, corn, avocado, and cilantro.
2. Toss gently to mix evenly.

Nutrition Information (per serving):

- Calories: 320
- Protein: 12g
- Carbohydrates: 50g
- Fat: 10g
- Fiber: 12g
- Sugar: 2g
- Portion Size: 1 serving

Turkey and Veggie Wrap

Ingredients:

- 4 whole wheat wraps
- 1 pound ground turkey, cooked
- 1 cup mixed bell peppers, sliced
- 1 cup lettuce, shredded
- 1/2 cup hummus

Instructions:

1. Lay out the wraps and spread hummus evenly.

2. Divide cooked ground turkey among the wraps.

3. Top with sliced bell peppers and shredded lettuce.

4. Roll the wraps tightly.

Nutrition Information (per serving):

- Calories: 380

- Protein: 25g

- Carbohydrates: 35g

- Fat: 16g

- Fiber: 8g

- Sugar: 4g

- Portion Size: 1 serving

Lentil Soup with Spinach

Ingredients:

- 1 cup dried green lentils, rinsed

- 1 onion, diced

- 2 carrots, diced

- 2 celery stalks, chopped

- 3 cloves garlic, minced

- 4 cups vegetable broth
- 2 cups fresh spinach
- 1 teaspoon cumin
- Salt and pepper to taste

Instructions:

1. In a pot, combine lentils, onion, carrots, celery, garlic, and vegetable broth.
2. Bring to a boil, then reduce heat and simmer until lentils are tender.
3. Stir in spinach, cumin, salt, and pepper.
4. Simmer until spinach is wilted.

Nutrition Information (per serving):

- Calories: 250
- Protein: 18g
- Carbohydrates: 40g
- Fat: 1g
- Fiber: 15g
- Sugar: 5g
- Portion Size: 1 serving

Shrimp and Vegetable Stir-Fry

Ingredients:

- 1 pound shrimp, peeled and deveined
- 2 cups broccoli florets
- 1 bell pepper, sliced
- 1 cup snap peas
- 3 tablespoons low-sodium soy sauce
- 1 tablespoon sesame oil
- 1 teaspoon ginger, grated
- 2 cloves garlic, minced

Instructions:

1. In a wok or skillet, heat sesame oil over medium-high heat.
2. Add shrimp and stir-fry until pink.
3. Add broccoli, bell pepper, snap peas, ginger, and garlic.
4. Stir in soy sauce and cook until vegetables are tender-crisp.

Nutrition Information (per serving):

- Calories: 280

- Protein: 25g

- Carbohydrates: 15g

- Fat: 12g

- Fiber: 5g

- Sugar: 6g

- Portion Size: 1 serving

Chickpea and Avocado Salad

Ingredients:

- 1 can chickpeas, drained and rinsed

- 1 avocado, diced

- 1 cup cherry tomatoes, halved

- 1/4 cup red onion, finely chopped

- 2 tablespoons fresh parsley, chopped

- 1 tablespoon olive oil

- 1 tablespoon balsamic vinegar

- Salt and pepper to taste

Instructions:

1. In a bowl, combine chickpeas, avocado, cherry tomatoes, red onion, and parsley.

2. Drizzle with olive oil and balsamic vinegar.

3. Season with salt and pepper, toss gently.

Nutrition Information (per serving):

- Calories: 320
- Protein: 10g
- Carbohydrates: 40g
- Fat: 16g
- Fiber: 12g
- Sugar: 5g
- Portion Size: 1 serving

Turkey and Sweet Potato Chili

Ingredients:

- 1 pound ground turkey
- 2 sweet potatoes, peeled and diced
- 1 can diced tomatoes
- 1 can black beans, drained and rinsed
- 1 onion, diced
- 3 cloves garlic, minced
- 2 tablespoons chili powder
- 1 teaspoon cumin
- Salt and pepper to taste

Instructions:

1. In a pot, brown ground turkey with onions and garlic.
2. Add sweet potatoes, diced tomatoes, black beans, chili powder, cumin, salt, and pepper.
3. Simmer until sweet potatoes are tender.

Nutrition Information (per serving):

- Calories: 380
- Protein: 25g
- Carbohydrates: 40g
- Fat: 14g
- Fiber: 10g
- Sugar: 8g
- Portion Size: 1 serving

Caprese Salad with Balsamic Glaze

Ingredients:

- 4 large tomatoes, sliced
- 1 ball fresh mozzarella, sliced
- 1/4 cup fresh basil leaves
- 2 tablespoons balsamic glaze
- Salt and pepper to taste

Instructions:

1. Arrange tomato and mozzarella slices on a plate.
2. Tuck fresh basil leaves between slices.
3. Drizzle with balsamic glaze and season with salt and pepper.

Nutrition Information (per serving):

- Calories: 250
- Protein: 12g
- Carbohydrates: 10g
- Fat: 18g
- Fiber: 2g
- Sugar: 5g
- Portion Size: 1 serving

Broccoli and Brown Rice Casserole

Ingredients:

- 2 cups broccoli florets
- 1 cup brown rice, cooked
- 1 cup cheddar cheese, shredded
- 1/2 cup plain Greek yogurt
- 1/4 cup milk

- 2 tablespoons whole wheat flour

- 1 teaspoon Dijon mustard

- Salt and pepper to taste

Instructions:

1. Steam broccoli until tender-crisp.

2. In a bowl, mix cooked brown rice, steamed broccoli, and half of the shredded cheddar.

3. In a separate bowl, whisk together Greek yogurt, milk, flour, Dijon mustard, salt, and pepper.

4. Pour the yogurt mixture over the rice and broccoli, mix well.

5. Transfer to a baking dish, top with the remaining cheddar, and bake until bubbly.

Nutrition Information (per serving):

- Calories: 300

- Protein: 15g

- Carbohydrates: 35g

- Fat: 12g

- Fiber: 5g

- Sugar: 3g

- Portion Size: 1 serving

Tofu and Vegetable Skewers

Ingredients:

- 1 block extra-firm tofu, cubed
- 2 bell peppers, cut into chunks
- 1 zucchini, sliced
- 1 red onion, cut into wedges
- 2 tablespoons soy sauce
- 1 tablespoon olive oil
- 1 teaspoon garlic powder
- 1 teaspoon smoked paprika

Instructions:

1. Preheat the grill or grill pan.
2. In a bowl, combine cubed tofu, bell peppers, zucchini, red onion, soy sauce, olive oil, garlic powder, and smoked paprika.
3. Thread the tofu and vegetables onto skewers.
4. Grill until tofu is golden and vegetables are tender.

Nutrition Information (per serving):

- Calories: 280
- Protein: 20g

- Carbohydrates: 15g

- Fat: 16g

- Fiber: 5g

- Sugar: 6g

- Portion Size: 1 serving

Mediterranean Quinoa Salad

Ingredients:

- 1 cup quinoa, cooked

- 1 cucumber, diced

- 1 cup cherry tomatoes, halved

- 1/2 cup Kalamata olives, sliced

- 1/4 cup red onion, finely chopped

- 1/3 cup feta cheese, crumbled

- 2 tablespoons olive oil

- 1 tablespoon red wine vinegar

- Fresh oregano, chopped

Instructions:

1. In a large bowl, combine cooked quinoa, cucumber, cherry tomatoes, Kalamata olives, red onion, and feta cheese.

2. Drizzle with olive oil and red wine vinegar.

3. Sprinkle with fresh oregano and toss gently.

Nutrition Information (per serving):

- Calories: 320
- Protein: 12g
- Carbohydrates: 40g
- Fat: 14g
- Fiber: 8g
- Sugar: 4g
- Portion Size: 1 serving

Zucchini Noodles with Pesto

Ingredients:

- 4 medium zucchinis, spiralized
- 1 cup cherry tomatoes, halved
- 1/2 cup pine nuts, toasted
- 1/2 cup fresh basil leaves
- 1/3 cup Parmesan cheese, grated
- 2 cloves garlic
- 1/2 cup extra-virgin olive oil
- Salt and pepper to taste

Instructions:

1. Spiralize zucchinis into noodles.
2. In a food processor, combine cherry tomatoes, toasted pine nuts, basil, Parmesan, and garlic.
3. While processing, slowly add olive oil until a smooth pesto forms.
4. Toss zucchini noodles with pesto, season with salt and pepper.

Nutrition Information (per serving):

- Calories: 290
- Protein: 8g
- Carbohydrates: 10g
- Fat: 25g
- Fiber: 4g
- Sugar: 5g
- Portion Size: 1 serving

Chicken and Vegetable Lettuce Wraps

Ingredients:

- 1 pound ground chicken
- 1 cup mushrooms, finely chopped
- 1 carrot, grated
- 1/2 cup water chestnuts, chopped
- 3 green onions, sliced
- 2 tablespoons soy sauce
- 1 tablespoon hoisin sauce
- 1 teaspoon sesame oil
- Iceberg lettuce leaves

Instructions:

1. In a skillet, brown ground chicken.
2. Add mushrooms, carrot, water chestnuts, and green onions.
3. Stir in soy sauce, hoisin sauce, and sesame oil.
4. Spoon mixture into lettuce leaves and serve.

Nutrition Information (per serving):

- Calories: 280

- Protein: 20g

- Carbohydrates: 15g

- Fat: 15g

- Fiber: 4g

- Sugar: 6g

- Portion Size: 1 serving

Cauliflower Fried Rice

Ingredients:

- 1 head cauliflower, grated

- 1 cup mixed vegetables (peas, carrots, corn)

- 2 eggs, beaten

- 3 tablespoons soy sauce

- 1 tablespoon sesame oil

- 1/2 cup green onions, chopped

- 1 teaspoon ginger, grated

Instructions:

1. In a large skillet, sauté cauliflower and mixed vegetables until tender.

2. Push vegetables to the side, pour beaten eggs into the skillet, and scramble.

3. Mix eggs with vegetables, then stir in soy sauce, sesame oil, green onions, and ginger.

Nutrition Information (per serving):

- Calories: 220
- Protein: 12g
- Carbohydrates: 20g
- Fat: 10g
- Fiber: 8g
- Sugar: 6g
- Portion Size: 1 serving

Greek Chicken Souvlaki

Ingredients:

- 1 pound chicken breast, cut into cubes
- 1/4 cup olive oil
- 2 tablespoons lemon juice
- 1 teaspoon dried oregano
- 2 cloves garlic, minced
- 1 cucumber, diced
- 1 cup cherry tomatoes, halved
- 1/2 cup feta cheese, crumbled

- Whole wheat pita bread

Instructions:

1. In a bowl, combine olive oil, lemon juice, oregano, and garlic.
2. Marinate chicken cubes in the mixture for at least 30 minutes.
3. Thread chicken onto skewers and grill until cooked.
4. Serve with diced cucumber, cherry tomatoes, feta, and whole wheat pita.

Nutrition Information (per serving):

- Calories: 340
- Protein: 25g
- Carbohydrates: 20g
- Fat: 18g
- Fiber: 4g
- Sugar: 6g
- Portion Size: 1 serving

Chapter 4: Dinner Recipes

In Chapter 4 of the "Simplest Type 2 Diabetes Cookbook for Beginners," we present a delightful array of Dinner Recipes crafted to make your evenings both delicious and nutritious.

Baked Salmon with Dill Sauce:

Ingredients:

- 4 salmon fillets
- 2 tablespoons olive oil
- 1 tablespoon fresh dill, chopped
- 1 lemon, sliced
- Salt and pepper to taste

Instructions:

1. Preheat the oven to 400°F (200°C).
2. Place salmon fillets on a baking sheet.
3. Drizzle with olive oil, sprinkle with salt, pepper, and chopped dill.
4. Top each fillet with lemon slices.

5. Bake for 15-20 minutes until salmon is cooked through.

6. Serve with a side of steamed vegetables.

Nutrition Information (per serving):

- Calories: 300

- Protein: 25g

- Carbohydrates: 0g

- Fat: 20g

- Fiber: 0g

- Sugar: 0g

- Portion Size: 1 fillet

Spaghetti Squash with Turkey Bolognese:

Ingredients:

- 1 spaghetti squash

- 1 lb ground turkey

- 1 onion, diced

- 2 cloves garlic, minced

- 1 can crushed tomatoes

- 1 teaspoon dried oregano
- Salt and pepper to taste

Instructions:

1. Cut the spaghetti squash in half, remove seeds, and roast until tender.
2. In a skillet, brown turkey over medium heat.
3. Add diced onions and garlic, cook until softened.
4. Stir in crushed tomatoes, oregano, salt, and pepper.
5. Simmer for 15-20 minutes.
6. Scrape the cooked spaghetti squash with a fork and top with turkey Bolognese.

Nutrition Information (per serving):

- Calories: 320
- Protein: 22g
- Carbohydrates: 25g
- Fat: 15g
- Fiber: 5g
- Sugar: 10g
- Portion Size: 1 cup

Lemon Herb Grilled Chicken:

Ingredients:

- 4 boneless, skinless chicken breasts
- 2 tablespoons olive oil
- 1 lemon, juiced
- 2 teaspoons dried herbs (rosemary, thyme, or oregano)
- Salt and pepper to taste

Instructions:

1. Preheat the grill to medium-high heat.
2. In a bowl, mix olive oil, lemon juice, dried herbs, salt, and pepper.
3. Marinate chicken breasts in the mixture for 30 minutes.
4. Grill chicken for 6-8 minutes per side until fully cooked.
5. Serve with a side of roasted vegetables.

Nutrition Information (per serving):

- Calories: 250
- Protein: 30g

- Carbohydrates: 2g

- Fat: 12g

- Fiber: 1g

- Sugar: 0g

- Portion Size: 1 breast

Eggplant and Tomato Stacks:

Ingredients:

- 1 large eggplant, sliced

- 4 large tomatoes, sliced

- 1 cup fresh mozzarella, sliced

- 1/4 cup fresh basil leaves

- Balsamic glaze for drizzling

- Salt and pepper to taste

Instructions:

1. Preheat the oven to 375°F (190°C).

2. Arrange eggplant and tomato slices on a baking sheet.

3. Sprinkle with salt and pepper, then roast for 15-20 minutes.

4. Assemble stacks by layering eggplant, tomato, and mozzarella.

5. Bake for an additional 10 minutes until cheese melts.

6. Garnish with fresh basil and drizzle with balsamic glaze.

Nutrition Information (per serving):

- Calories: 180
- Protein: 10g
- Carbohydrates: 15g
- Fat: 8g
- Fiber: 5g
- Sugar: 8g
- Portion Size: 1 stack

Blackened Tilapia with Mango Salsa:

Ingredients:

- 4 tilapia fillets
- 1 tablespoon blackened seasoning
- 1 tablespoon olive oil
- 1 mango, diced
- 1/2 red onion, finely chopped

- 1 jalapeño, minced
- Fresh cilantro, chopped
- Lime juice to taste
- Salt and pepper to taste

Instructions:

1. Rub tilapia fillets with blackened seasoning.
2. Heat olive oil in a skillet over medium-high heat.
3. Cook tilapia for 3-4 minutes per side until blackened and cooked through.
4. In a bowl, combine mango, red onion, jalapeño, cilantro, lime juice, salt, and pepper.
5. Serve blackened tilapia topped with mango salsa.

Nutrition Information (per serving):

- Calories: 220
- Protein: 25g
- Carbohydrates: 15g
- Fat: 8g
- Fiber: 3g
- Sugar: 10g
- Portion Size: 1 fillet with salsa

Stuffed Bell Peppers with Quinoa:

Ingredients:

- 4 large bell peppers, halved and seeds removed
- 1 cup cooked quinoa
- 1 lb lean ground beef or turkey
- 1 onion, diced
- 1 can black beans, drained and rinsed
- 1 cup diced tomatoes
- 1 cup shredded cheddar cheese
- 1 teaspoon cumin
- Salt and pepper to taste

Instructions:

1. Preheat the oven to 375°F (190°C).
2. In a skillet, brown ground meat and onions.
3. Add cooked quinoa, black beans, tomatoes, cumin, salt, and pepper.
4. Spoon the mixture into halved bell peppers.
5. Top with shredded cheese and bake for 25-30 minutes.
6. Garnish with fresh cilantro before serving.

Nutrition Information (per serving):

- Calories: 320
- Protein: 25g
- Carbohydrates: 30g
- Fat: 12g
- Fiber: 7g
- Sugar: 5g
- Portion Size: 1 stuffed pepper

Teriyaki Tofu Stir-Fry:

Ingredients:

- 1 block extra-firm tofu, cubed
- 2 cups broccoli florets
- 1 red bell pepper, sliced
- 1 carrot, julienned
- 1/2 cup snap peas
- 1/4 cup low-sodium teriyaki sauce
- 2 tablespoons sesame oil
- 2 cloves garlic, minced
- 1 teaspoon ginger, grated
- Sesame seeds for garnish

Instructions:

1. Press tofu to remove excess water, then cube it.
2. In a wok or skillet, heat sesame oil over medium-high heat.
3. Add tofu and stir-fry until golden brown.
4. Add garlic and ginger, followed by broccoli, bell pepper, carrot, and snap peas.
5. Pour teriyaki sauce over the stir-fry and toss until vegetables are tender.
6. Garnish with sesame seeds before serving.

Nutrition Information (per serving):

- Calories: 240
- Protein: 15g
- Carbohydrates: 20g
- Fat: 12g
- Fiber: 5g
- Sugar: 8g
- Portion Size: 1 cup

Cilantro Lime Shrimp Skewers:

Ingredients:

- 1 lb large shrimp, peeled and deveined
- Zest and juice of 2 limes
- 2 tablespoons fresh cilantro, chopped
- 1 tablespoon olive oil
- 2 cloves garlic, minced
- 1 teaspoon cumin
- Salt and pepper to taste
- Wooden skewers, soaked in water

Instructions:

1. In a bowl, mix lime zest, lime juice, cilantro, olive oil, garlic, cumin, salt, and pepper.
2. Thread shrimp onto skewers and brush with the marinade.
3. Grill skewers over medium-high heat for 2-3 minutes per side.
4. Serve with additional lime wedges.

Nutrition Information (per serving):

- Calories: 180

- Protein: 20g

- Carbohydrates: 2g

- Fat: 10g

- Fiber: 0g

- Sugar: 0g

- Portion Size: 4 skewers

Sweet Potato and Chickpea Curry:

Ingredients:

- 2 sweet potatoes, peeled and diced

- 1 can chickpeas, drained and rinsed

- 1 onion, diced

- 2 cloves garlic, minced

- 1 can coconut milk

- 2 tablespoons curry powder

- 1 teaspoon turmeric

- Salt and pepper to taste

- Fresh cilantro for garnish

Instructions:

1. In a pot, sauté onions and garlic until softened.

2. Add sweet potatoes, chickpeas, curry powder, turmeric, salt, and pepper.

3. Pour in coconut milk and bring to a simmer.

4. Cook until sweet potatoes are tender.

5. Garnish with fresh cilantro before serving.

Nutrition Information (per serving):

- Calories: 280
- Protein: 8g
- Carbohydrates: 35g
- Fat: 12g
- Fiber: 7g
- Sugar: 8g
- Portion Size: 1 cup

Grilled Portobello Mushrooms with Garlic:

Ingredients:

- 4 large Portobello mushrooms
- 3 tablespoons olive oil
- 4 cloves garlic, minced

- 2 tablespoons balsamic vinegar

- Salt and pepper to taste

- Fresh parsley for garnish

Instructions:

1. Clean mushrooms and remove stems.
2. In a bowl, mix olive oil, minced garlic, balsamic vinegar, salt, and pepper.
3. Brush the mixture over both sides of the mushrooms.
4. Grill mushrooms for 4-5 minutes per side.
5. Garnish with fresh parsley before serving.

Nutrition Information (per serving):

- Calories: 120

- Protein: 4g

- Carbohydrates: 8g

- Fat: 9g

- Fiber: 2g

- Sugar: 3g

- Portion Size: 1 mushroom

Turkey and Vegetable Casserole:

Ingredients:

- 1 lb ground turkey
- 1 onion, diced
- 2 bell peppers, diced
- 2 zucchinis, sliced
- 1 cup cherry tomatoes, halved
- 1 cup quinoa, cooked
- 1 cup low-sodium tomato sauce
- 1 teaspoon Italian seasoning
- Salt and pepper to taste
- 1 cup shredded mozzarella cheese

Instructions:

1. Preheat the oven to 375°F (190°C).
2. In a skillet, brown ground turkey with onions.
3. Add bell peppers, zucchinis, and cherry tomatoes, cook until vegetables are tender.
4. Stir in cooked quinoa, tomato sauce, Italian seasoning, salt, and pepper.
5. Transfer the mixture to a baking dish and top with shredded mozzarella.

6. Bake for 20-25 minutes until cheese is bubbly and golden.

Nutrition Information (per serving):

- Calories: 320
- Protein: 25g
- Carbohydrates: 30g
- Fat: 12g
- Fiber: 5g
- Sugar: 8g
- Portion Size: 1 cup

Lemon Garlic Butter Shrimp:

Ingredients:

- 1 lb large shrimp, peeled and deveined
- 3 tablespoons unsalted butter
- 4 cloves garlic, minced
- Zest and juice of 1 lemon
- 1 teaspoon paprika
- Salt and pepper to taste
- Fresh parsley for garnish

Instructions:

1. In a skillet, melt butter over medium heat.

2. Add minced garlic and cook until fragrant.

3. Stir in shrimp, lemon zest, lemon juice, paprika, salt, and pepper.

4. Cook shrimp for 2-3 minutes per side until pink and opaque.

5. Garnish with fresh parsley before serving.

Nutrition Information (per serving):

- Calories: 220
- Protein: 20g
- Carbohydrates: 2g
- Fat: 14g
- Fiber: 0g
- Sugar: 0g
- Portion Size: 1 cup

Ratatouille with Herbed Quinoa:

Ingredients:

- 1 eggplant, diced
- 2 zucchinis, sliced

- 1 bell pepper, diced
- 1 onion, diced
- 2 tomatoes, diced
- 3 cloves garlic, minced
- 2 tablespoons olive oil
- 1 teaspoon dried thyme
- 1 teaspoon dried rosemary
- Salt and pepper to taste
- 1 cup cooked quinoa

Instructions:

1. Preheat the oven to 375°F (190°C).
2. In a large baking dish, toss eggplant, zucchinis, bell pepper, onion, tomatoes, and garlic.
3. Drizzle with olive oil, sprinkle with thyme, rosemary, salt, and pepper.
4. Roast for 30-40 minutes until vegetables are tender.
5. Serve over a bed of herbed quinoa.

Nutrition Information (per serving):

- Calories: 250
- Protein: 8g

- Carbohydrates: 35g
- Fat: 10g
- Fiber: 8g
- Sugar: 10g
- Portion Size: 1 cup

Baked Chicken Breast with Rosemary:

Ingredients:

- 4 boneless, skinless chicken breasts
- 2 tablespoons olive oil
- 2 teaspoons fresh rosemary, chopped
- 2 cloves garlic, minced
- 1 lemon, sliced
- Salt and pepper to taste

Instructions:

1. Preheat the oven to 400°F (200°C).
2. Rub chicken breasts with olive oil, chopped rosemary, minced garlic, salt, and pepper.

3. Place chicken on a baking sheet and top with lemon slices.

4. Bake for 25-30 minutes until chicken is cooked through.

5. Serve with a side of roasted vegetables.

Nutrition Information (per serving):

- Calories: 280
- Protein: 30g
- Carbohydrates: 1g
- Fat: 16g
- Fiber: 0g
- Sugar: 0g
- Portion Size: 1 breast

Mexican Cauliflower Rice Bowl:

Ingredients:

- 1 head cauliflower, grated
- 1 lb lean ground beef or turkey
- 1 onion, diced
- 1 bell pepper, diced
- 1 cup corn kernels

- 1 cup black beans, drained and rinsed
- 1 tablespoon chili powder
- 1 teaspoon cumin
- Salt and pepper to taste
- Fresh cilantro for garnish

Instructions:

1. In a large skillet, brown ground meat with diced onions.
2. Add grated cauliflower, bell pepper, corn, black beans, chili powder, cumin, salt, and pepper.
3. Cook until cauliflower is tender and flavors meld.
4. Serve in bowls, garnished with fresh cilantro.

Nutrition Information (per serving):

- Calories: 290
- Protein: 25g
- Carbohydrates: 20g
- Fat: 12g
- Fiber: 8g
- Sugar: 5g
- Portion Size: 1 bowl

Chapter 5: Snacks and Appetizers

These recipes are crafted to bring together the perfect balance of flavors, providing you with wholesome choices for every snacking occasion.

Guacamole with Veggie Sticks

Ingredients:

- 2 ripe avocados
- 1 medium tomato, diced
- 1/4 cup red onion, finely chopped
- 1 clove garlic, minced
- 1 lime, juiced
- Salt and pepper to taste
- Assorted veggie sticks (carrots, celery, bell peppers)

Instructions:

1. Mash the avocados in a bowl.
2. Add diced tomato, chopped red onion, minced garlic, and lime juice.
3. Season with salt and pepper to taste.

4. Mix well and serve with veggie sticks.

Nutrition Information (per serving):

- Calories: 120
- Protein: 2g
- Carbohydrates: 10g
- Fat: 9g
- Fiber: 6g
- Sugar: 2g
- Portion size: 1/2 cup guacamole with veggie sticks

Greek Yogurt and Berry Parfait

Ingredients:

- 1 cup Greek yogurt
- 1/2 cup mixed berries (strawberries, blueberries, raspberries)
- 2 tablespoons honey
- Granola (optional)

Instructions:

1. In a glass or bowl, layer Greek yogurt.
2. Add a layer of mixed berries.

3. Drizzle with honey.

4. Repeat the layers.

5. Top with granola if desired.

Nutrition Information (per serving):

- Calories: 200

- Protein: 15g

- Carbohydrates: 25g

- Fat: 6g

- Fiber: 3g

- Sugar: 18g

- Portion size: 1 cup parfait

Hummus and Whole Wheat Pita

Ingredients:

- 1 cup hummus

- Whole wheat pita, cut into triangles

Instructions:

1. Spoon hummus into a serving bowl.

2. Serve with whole wheat pita triangles.

Nutrition Information (per serving):

- Calories: 180
- Protein: 8g
- Carbohydrates: 22g
- Fat: 8g
- Fiber: 6g
- Sugar: 1g
- Portion size: 1/2 cup hummus with 4 pita triangles

Cucumber and Tuna Bites

Ingredients:

- 1 cucumber, sliced
- 1 can tuna, drained
- 2 tablespoons mayonnaise
- 1 tablespoon Dijon mustard
- Salt and pepper to taste

Instructions:

1. In a bowl, mix tuna, mayonnaise, Dijon mustard, salt, and pepper.
2. Place a spoonful of tuna mixture on each cucumber slice.

3. Garnish with fresh herbs if desired.

Nutrition Information (per serving):

- Calories: 90
- Protein: 15g
- Carbohydrates: 2g
- Fat: 3g
- Fiber: 1g
- Sugar: 0g
- Portion size: 4 cucumber and tuna bites

Edamame with Sea Salt

Ingredients:

- 1 cup edamame (in pods)
- Sea salt to taste

Instructions:

1. Boil or steam edamame according to package instructions.
2. Sprinkle with sea salt.
3. Toss to coat and serve.

Nutrition Information (per serving):

- Calories: 120
- Protein: 11g
- Carbohydrates: 9g
- Fat: 5g
- Fiber: 4g
- Sugar: 3g
- Portion size: 1 cup edamame

Almond and Cranberry Trail Mix

Ingredients:

- 1/2 cup almonds
- 1/4 cup dried cranberries
- 1/4 cup pumpkin seeds
- 1/4 cup dark chocolate chips (optional)

Instructions:

1. Mix almonds, dried cranberries, pumpkin seeds, and dark chocolate chips.
2. Portion into snack-sized bags for easy grab-and-go.

Nutrition Information (per serving):

- Calories: 180

- Protein: 5g

- Carbohydrates: 15g

- Fat: 12g

- Fiber: 3g

- Sugar: 8g

- Portion size: 1/4 cup trail mix

Caprese Skewers with Cherry Tomatoes

Ingredients:

- Cherry tomatoes

- Fresh mozzarella balls

- Basil leaves

- Balsamic glaze

Instructions:

1. Thread a cherry tomato, mozzarella ball, and basil leaf onto skewers.

2. Arrange on a serving platter.

3. Drizzle with balsamic glaze before serving.

Nutrition Information (per serving):

- Calories: 120
- Protein: 8g
- Carbohydrates: 4g
- Fat: 8g
- Fiber: 1g
- Sugar: 2g
- Portion size: 4 skewers

Apple Slices with Peanut Butter

Ingredients:

- 2 apples, sliced
- 1/4 cup natural peanut butter

Instructions:

1. Spread peanut butter on apple slices.
2. Arrange on a plate and serve.

Nutrition Information (per serving):

- Calories: 200

- Protein: 6g

- Carbohydrates: 25g

- Fat: 10g

- Fiber: 6g

- Sugar: 18g

- Portion size: 1 apple with peanut butter

Cottage Cheese and Pineapple Cups

Ingredients:

- 1 cup low-fat cottage cheese
- 1 cup fresh pineapple chunks

Instructions:

1. Divide cottage cheese into serving cups.
2. Top with fresh pineapple chunks.

Nutrition Information (per serving):

- Calories: 180
- Protein: 20g
- Carbohydrates: 25g
- Fat: 2g
- Fiber: 3g

- Sugar: 18g
- Portion size: 1 cup cottage cheese with pineapple

Roasted Red Pepper and Feta Dip

Ingredients:

- 1 cup roasted red peppers (from a jar), drained
- 1/2 cup feta cheese
- 1 clove garlic
- 2 tablespoons olive oil
- Salt and pepper to taste

Instructions:

1. In a food processor, blend roasted red peppers, feta, garlic, and olive oil until smooth.
2. Season with salt and pepper.
3. Serve with whole grain crackers or vegetable sticks.

Nutrition Information (per serving):

- Calories: 120
- Protein: 4g
- Carbohydrates: 5g
- Fat: 10g

- Fiber: 2g
- Sugar: 3g
- Portion size: 1/4 cup dip

Hard-Boiled Egg with Mustard

Ingredients:

- 2 hard-boiled eggs
- Mustard for dipping

Instructions:

1. Peel the hard-boiled eggs.
2. Serve with a side of mustard for dipping.

Nutrition Information (per serving):

- Calories: 140
- Protein: 12g
- Carbohydrates: 2g
- Fat: 10g
- Fiber: 0g
- Sugar: 0g
- Portion size: 2 eggs with mustard

Avocado and Tomato Salsa

Ingredients:

- 2 avocados, diced
- 1 cup cherry tomatoes, halved
- 1/4 cup red onion, finely chopped
- 1/4 cup fresh cilantro, chopped
- 1 lime, juiced
- Salt and pepper to taste

Instructions:

1. In a bowl, combine diced avocados, cherry tomatoes, red onion, cilantro, and lime juice.
2. Season with salt and pepper.
3. Mix gently and serve with whole grain tortilla chips.

Nutrition Information (per serving):

- Calories: 160
- Protein: 2g
- Carbohydrates: 12g
- Fat: 14g
- Fiber: 7g
- Sugar: 2g

- Portion size: 1/2 cup salsa with chips

Spinach and Artichoke Dip

Ingredients:

- 1 cup frozen spinach, thawed and drained
- 1 cup canned artichoke hearts, chopped
- 1/2 cup Greek yogurt
- 1/4 cup mayonnaise
- 1/4 cup grated Parmesan cheese
- 1 clove garlic, minced

Instructions:

1. Preheat oven to 350°F (175°C).
2. In a bowl, mix spinach, artichoke hearts, Greek yogurt, mayonnaise, Parmesan cheese, and minced garlic.
3. Transfer to a baking dish and bake for 20 minutes or until bubbly.
4. Serve with vegetable sticks.

Nutrition Information (per serving):

- Calories: 150

- Protein: 6g

- Carbohydrates: 8g

- Fat: 10g

- Fiber: 3g

- Sugar: 2g

- Portion size: 1/4 cup dip with veggies

Mixed Nuts and Seeds

Ingredients:

- 1/2 cup mixed nuts (almonds, walnuts, cashews)

- 2 tablespoons mixed seeds (pumpkin, sunflower)

Instructions:

1. Combine mixed nuts and seeds in a bowl.

2. Toss together and portion into snack-sized bags.

Nutrition Information (per serving):

- Calories: 200

- Protein: 6g

- Carbohydrates: 8g

- Fat: 18g

- Fiber: 4g

- Sugar: 1g

- Portion size: 1/4 cup nut and seed mix

Stuffed Mini Bell Peppers

Ingredients:

- 10 mini bell peppers

- 1 cup cream cheese, softened

- 1/4 cup green onions, chopped

- 1/4 cup shredded cheddar cheese

Instructions:

1. Cut mini bell peppers in half lengthwise and remove seeds.

2. In a bowl, mix cream cheese and green onions.

3. Stuff each pepper half with the cream cheese mixture.

4. Top with shredded cheddar cheese.

Nutrition Information (per serving):

- Calories: 120

- Protein: 4g

- Carbohydrates: 5g

- Fat: 10g

- Fiber: 1g

- Sugar: 3g

- Portion size: 5 stuffed pepper halves

Chapter 6: Desserts

In this chapter, we delve into delectable desserts that not only satisfy your sweet cravings but also align with a diabetes-friendly lifestyle.

Berry and Greek Yogurt Popsicles

Ingredients:

- 1 cup mixed berries (strawberries, blueberries, raspberries)
- 1 cup Greek yogurt (low-fat or non-fat)
- 2 tablespoons honey
- 1 teaspoon vanilla extract

Instructions:

1. Blend berries, Greek yogurt, honey, and vanilla extract until smooth.
2. Pour the mixture into popsicle molds.
3. Freeze for at least 4 hours or until firm.
4. Run molds under warm water to release popsicles.

Nutrition Information (per serving):

- Calories: 80
- Protein: 4g
- Carbohydrates: 15g
- Fat: 1g
- Fiber: 2g
- Sugar: 11g
- Portion Size: 1 popsicle

Dark Chocolate-Dipped Strawberries

Ingredients:

- 1 cup fresh strawberries
- 3 oz dark chocolate (70% cocoa or higher)

Instructions:

1. Melt dark chocolate in a heatproof bowl.
2. Dip each strawberry into the melted chocolate.
3. Place on parchment paper and refrigerate until chocolate hardens.

Nutrition Information (per serving):

- Calories: 60

- Protein: 1g

- Carbohydrates: 10g

- Fat: 3g

- Fiber: 2g

- Sugar: 5g

- Portion Size: 4 strawberries

Baked Apples with Cinnamon

Ingredients:

- 2 apples, cored and halved

- 1 teaspoon cinnamon

- 1 tablespoon melted butter (or coconut oil)

Instructions:

1. Preheat the oven to 375°F (190°C).

2. Place apple halves on a baking sheet.

3. Mix cinnamon with melted butter and brush over apples.

4. Bake for 25-30 minutes until apples are tender.

Nutrition Information (per serving):

- Calories: 120

- Protein: 1g

- Carbohydrates: 28g

- Fat: 3g

- Fiber: 5g

- Sugar: 20g

- Portion Size: 1 apple half

Sugar-Free Mango Sorbet

Ingredients:

- 2 cups frozen mango chunks

- 1/4 cup water

- 1 tablespoon lime juice

- 1-2 tablespoons sugar substitute (optional)

Instructions:

1. Blend frozen mango, water, lime juice, and sugar substitute until smooth.

2. Transfer to a container and freeze for at least 2 hours.

Nutrition Information (per serving):

- Calories: 90

- Protein: 1g

- Carbohydrates: 22g

- Fat: 0g

- Fiber: 3g

- Sugar: 18g

- Portion Size: 1/2 cup

Almond Flour Chocolate Chip Cookies

Ingredients:

- 1 cup almond flour

- 1/4 cup coconut oil (melted)

- 1/4 cup sugar substitute

- 1 egg

- 1/2 teaspoon vanilla extract

- 1/4 teaspoon baking soda

- 1/4 cup sugar-free chocolate chips

Instructions:

1. Preheat the oven to 350°F (175°C).

2. In a bowl, mix almond flour, melted coconut oil, sugar substitute, egg, vanilla extract, and baking soda.

3. Fold in sugar-free chocolate chips.

4. Drop spoonfuls of dough onto a baking sheet and bake for 10-12 minutes.

Nutrition Information (per serving):

- Calories: 90
- Protein: 2g
- Carbohydrates: 5g
- Fat: 7g
- Fiber: 1g
- Sugar: 1g
- Portion Size: 2 cookies

Chia Seed Chocolate Pudding

Ingredients:

- 1/4 cup chia seeds
- 1 cup unsweetened almond milk
- 2 tablespoons cocoa powder
- 1-2 tablespoons sugar substitute

- 1/2 teaspoon vanilla extract

Instructions:

1. In a bowl, whisk together chia seeds, almond milk, cocoa powder, sugar substitute, and vanilla extract.
2. Refrigerate for at least 4 hours or overnight, stirring occasionally.

Nutrition Information (per serving):

- Calories: 80
- Protein: 3g
- Carbohydrates: 9g
- Fat: 4g
- Fiber: 6g
- Sugar: 0g
- Portion Size: 1/2 cup

Grilled Peaches with Honey

Ingredients:

- 2 peaches, halved and pitted
- 1 tablespoon honey
- 1/2 teaspoon cinnamon

Instructions:

1. Preheat the grill to medium-high heat.
2. Grill peach halves for 2-3 minutes per side.
3. Drizzle honey and sprinkle cinnamon over grilled peaches.

Nutrition Information (per serving):

- Calories: 60
- Protein: 1g
- Carbohydrates: 15g
- Fat: 0g
- Fiber: 2g
- Sugar: 12g
- Portion Size: 1 peach half

Vanilla Chia Seed Pudding

Ingredients:

- 1/4 cup chia seeds
- 1 cup unsweetened vanilla almond milk
- 1-2 tablespoons sugar substitute
- 1/2 teaspoon vanilla extract
- Fresh berries for topping

Instructions:

1. Mix chia seeds, almond milk, sugar substitute, and vanilla extract in a bowl.
2. Refrigerate for at least 3 hours or overnight.
3. Top with fresh berries before serving.

Nutrition Information (per serving):

- Calories: 70
- Protein: 3g
- Carbohydrates: 9g
- Fat: 3g
- Fiber: 5g
- Sugar: 1g
- Portion Size: 1/2 cup

Lemon Blueberry Muffins (Low-Sugar)

Ingredients:

- 1 cup almond flour
- 1/4 cup coconut flour
- 1/4 cup sugar substitute

- 1 teaspoon baking powder
- 1/4 teaspoon salt
- 1/4 cup melted coconut oil
- 3 large eggs
- 1/4 cup unsweetened almond milk
- 1 teaspoon vanilla extract
- 1 cup fresh blueberries
- Zest of 1 lemon

Instructions:

1. Preheat the oven to 350°F (175°C) and line a muffin tin with paper liners.
2. In a bowl, combine almond flour, coconut flour, sugar substitute, baking powder, and salt.
3. In another bowl, whisk together melted coconut oil, eggs, almond milk, and vanilla extract.
4. Add wet ingredients to the dry ingredients and mix until well combined.
5. Gently fold in blueberries and lemon zest.
6. Spoon batter into muffin cups and bake for 20-25 minutes.

Nutrition Information (per serving):

- Calories: 120
- Protein: 4g
- Carbohydrates: 8g
- Fat: 9g
- Fiber: 3g
- Sugar: 3g
- Portion Size: 1 muffin

Avocado Chocolate Mousse

Ingredients:

- 2 ripe avocados
- 1/4 cup cocoa powder
- 1/4 cup almond milk
- 1/4 cup sugar substitute
- 1 teaspoon vanilla extract
- Pinch of salt

Instructions:

1. Blend avocados, cocoa powder, almond milk, sugar substitute, vanilla extract, and salt until smooth.
2. Refrigerate for at least 2 hours before serving.

Nutrition Information (per serving):

- Calories: 100
- Protein: 2g
- Carbohydrates: 7g
- Fat: 8g
- Fiber: 5g
- Sugar: 1g
- Portion Size: 1/2 cup

Pumpkin Spice Energy Bites

Ingredients:

- 1 cup rolled oats
- 1/2 cup pumpkin puree
- 1/4 cup almond butter
- 1/4 cup ground flaxseed
- 1/4 cup chopped walnuts
- 2 tablespoons honey
- 1 teaspoon pumpkin spice
- 1/2 teaspoon vanilla extract

Instructions:

1. In a bowl, mix rolled oats, pumpkin puree, almond butter, flaxseed, walnuts, honey, pumpkin spice, and vanilla extract.

2. Roll into bite-sized balls and refrigerate for at least 30 minutes.

Nutrition Information (per serving):

- Calories: 90
- Protein: 3g
- Carbohydrates: 10g
- Fat: 5g
- Fiber: 2g
- Sugar: 3g
- Portion Size: 2 energy bites

Mixed Berry Crisp

Ingredients:

- 2 cups mixed berries (strawberries, blueberries, raspberries)
- 1 tablespoon lemon juice
- 1/4 cup rolled oats

- 2 tablespoons almond flour
- 1 tablespoon coconut oil (melted)
- 1 tablespoon honey
- 1/2 teaspoon cinnamon

Instructions:

1. Preheat the oven to 350°F (175°C).
2. Toss mixed berries with lemon juice and place in a baking dish.
3. In a bowl, mix rolled oats, almond flour, melted coconut oil, honey, and cinnamon.
4. Sprinkle the oat mixture over the berries and bake for 25-30 minutes.

Nutrition Information (per serving):

- Calories: 120
- Protein: 2g
- Carbohydrates: 20g
- Fat: 5g
- Fiber: 5g
- Sugar: 10g
- Portion Size: 1/2 cup

Coconut Milk Rice Pudding

Ingredients:

- 1/2 cup Arborio rice
- 2 cups light coconut milk
- 1/4 cup sugar substitute
- 1/2 teaspoon vanilla extract
- Pinch of salt
- Ground cinnamon for garnish

Instructions:

1. In a saucepan, combine rice, coconut milk, sugar substitute, vanilla extract, and salt.
2. Bring to a simmer, then reduce heat and cook until rice is tender.
3. Remove from heat and let it cool. Garnish with ground cinnamon before serving.

Nutrition Information (per serving):

- Calories: 150
- Protein: 2g
- Carbohydrates: 25g
- Fat: 5g

- Fiber: 1g

- Sugar: 0g

- Portion Size: 1/2 cup

Raspberry Almond Tarts

Ingredients:

- 1 cup almond flour

- 2 tablespoons coconut oil (melted)

- 1 tablespoon honey

- 1/2 teaspoon almond extract

- 1/2 cup fresh raspberries

Instructions:

1. Preheat the oven to 350°F (175°C).

2. In a bowl, combine almond flour, melted coconut oil, honey, and almond extract.

3. Press the mixture into tartlet pans to create crusts.

4. Bake for 10-12 minutes until golden brown.

5. Allow the crusts to cool, then fill each with fresh raspberries.

Nutrition Information (per serving):

- Calories: 110
- Protein: 3g
- Carbohydrates: 8g
- Fat: 8g
- Fiber: 2g
- Sugar: 4g
- Portion Size: 1 tart

Banana Walnut Muffins (No Added Sugar)

Ingredients:

- 1 cup almond flour
- 1/4 cup coconut flour
- 1 teaspoon baking powder
- 1/2 teaspoon baking soda
- 1/4 teaspoon salt
- 2 ripe bananas, mashed
- 1/4 cup melted coconut oil
- 2 large eggs
- 1/2 cup chopped walnuts

Instructions:

1. Preheat the oven to 350°F (175°C) and line a muffin tin with paper liners.
2. In a bowl, combine almond flour, coconut flour, baking powder, baking soda, and salt.
3. In another bowl, mix mashed bananas, melted coconut oil, and eggs.
4. Add wet ingredients to dry ingredients and stir until just combined.
5. Fold in chopped walnuts.
6. Spoon batter into muffin cups and bake for 20-25 minutes.

Nutrition Information (per serving):

- Calories: 130
- Protein: 4g
- Carbohydrates: 10g
- Fat: 9g
- Fiber: 3g
- Sugar: 3g
- Portion Size: 1 muffin

Chapter 7: Smoothies

In Chapter 7, we dive into a symphony of smoothie recipes that not only tantalize your taste buds but also align with your diabetes-friendly diet.

Green Detox Smoothie

Ingredients:

- 1 cup kale leaves, stems removed
- 1/2 cucumber, peeled and sliced
- 1 green apple, cored and chopped
- 1/2 lemon, juiced
- 1 cup water
- Ice cubes (optional)

Instructions:

1. Place kale, cucumber, apple, and lemon juice in a blender.
2. Add water and blend until smooth.
3. If desired, add ice cubes and blend again.
4. Pour into a glass and enjoy!

Nutrition Information (per serving):

- Calories: 90
- Protein: 2g
- Carbohydrates: 22g
- Fat: 0.5g
- Fiber: 5g
- Sugar: 12g
- Portion Size: 1 smoothie

Berry Blast Smoothie

Ingredients:

- 1 cup mixed berries (strawberries, blueberries, raspberries)
- 1/2 banana
- 1/2 cup plain Greek yogurt
- 1 tablespoon chia seeds
- 1 cup almond milk
- Ice cubes (optional)

Instructions:

1. Combine berries, banana, Greek yogurt, chia seeds, and almond milk in a blender.

2. Blend until smooth.

3. Add ice cubes if desired and blend again.

4. Pour into a glass and savor the berry goodness!

Nutrition Information (per serving):

- Calories: 120

- Protein: 6g

- Carbohydrates: 18g

- Fat: 3.5g

- Fiber: 5g

- Sugar: 10g

- Portion Size: 1 smoothie

Mango and Pineapple Paradise

Ingredients:

- 1 cup fresh mango chunks

- 1/2 cup pineapple chunks

- 1/2 banana

- 1/2 cup coconut water

- 1 tablespoon flaxseeds

- Ice cubes (optional)

Instructions:

1. Combine mango, pineapple, banana, coconut water, and flaxseeds in a blender.

2. Blend until smooth.

3. Add ice cubes if desired and blend again.

4. Pour into a glass and transport yourself to a tropical paradise!

Nutrition Information (per serving):

- Calories: 130

- Protein: 2g

- Carbohydrates: 30g

- Fat: 2g

- Fiber: 4g

- Sugar: 20g

- Portion Size: 1 smoothie

Spinach and Banana Delight

Ingredients:

- 2 cups fresh spinach leaves

- 1 banana

- 1/2 cup plain yogurt

- 1 tablespoon almond butter
- 1/2 teaspoon honey
- 1 cup water
- Ice cubes (optional)

Instructions:

1. Combine spinach, banana, yogurt, almond butter, honey, and water in a blender.
2. Blend until smooth.
3. If desired, add ice cubes and blend again.
4. Pour into a glass and relish the delightful combination.

Nutrition Information (per serving):

- Calories: 150
- Protein: 5g
- Carbohydrates: 20g
- Fat: 6g
- Fiber: 4g
- Sugar: 10g
- Portion Size: 1 smoothie

Antioxidant-Rich Blueberry Smoothie

Ingredients:

- 1 cup blueberries
- 1/2 cup spinach
- 1/2 cup kale
- 1/2 cup Greek yogurt
- 1 tablespoon hemp seeds
- 1 cup unsweetened almond milk
- Ice cubes (optional)

Instructions:

1. Combine blueberries, spinach, kale, Greek yogurt, hemp seeds, and almond milk in a blender.
2. Blend until smooth.
3. Add ice cubes if desired and blend again.
4. Pour into a glass and enjoy the antioxidant boost!

Nutrition Information (per serving):

- Calories: 120
- Protein: 6g
- Carbohydrates: 15g

- Fat: 4.5g
- Fiber: 4g
- Sugar: 8g
- Portion Size: 1 smoothie

Peanut Butter and Banana Protein Shake

Ingredients:

- 1 banana
- 2 tablespoons peanut butter
- 1/2 cup plain Greek yogurt
- 1 scoop vanilla protein powder
- 1 cup milk (dairy or plant-based)
- Ice cubes (optional)

Instructions:

1. Combine banana, peanut butter, Greek yogurt, protein powder, and milk in a blender.
2. Blend until smooth.
3. If desired, add ice cubes and blend again.

4. Pour into a glass and relish the protein-packed goodness.

Nutrition Information (per serving):

- Calories: 280
- Protein: 25g
- Carbohydrates: 20g
- Fat: 12g
- Fiber: 3g
- Sugar: 12g
- Portion Size: 1 smoothie

Citrus Burst Smoothie

Ingredients:

- 1 orange, peeled and segmented
- 1/2 grapefruit, peeled and segmented
- 1/2 cup Greek yogurt
- 1 tablespoon chia seeds
- 1 cup coconut water
- Ice cubes (optional)

Instructions:

1. Combine orange segments, grapefruit segments, Greek yogurt, chia seeds, and coconut water in a blender.
2. Blend until smooth.
3. Add ice cubes if desired and blend again.
4. Pour into a glass and experience the burst of citrusy freshness.

Nutrition Information (per serving):

- Calories: 140
- Protein: 5g
- Carbohydrates: 25g
- Fat: 3g
- Fiber: 6g
- Sugar: 15g
- Portion Size: 1 smoothie

Kale and Kiwi Elixir

Ingredients:

- 1 cup kale leaves, stems removed
- 2 kiwis, peeled and sliced

- 1/2 banana
- 1 tablespoon flaxseeds
- 1 cup green tea, chilled
- Ice cubes (optional)

Instructions:

1. Combine kale, kiwi, banana, flaxseeds, and chilled green tea in a blender.
2. Blend until smooth.
3. If desired, add ice cubes and blend again.
4. Pour into a glass and savor the elixir of health.

Nutrition Information (per serving):

- Calories: 110
- Protein: 4g
- Carbohydrates: 20g
- Fat: 3.5g
- Fiber: 5g
- Sugar: 10g
- Portion Size: 1 smoothie

Almond Joy Smoothie

Ingredients:

- 1/2 cup almonds, soaked and peeled
- 1 banana
- 2 tablespoons shredded coconut
- 1 tablespoon cocoa powder
- 1 cup almond milk
- Ice cubes (optional)

Instructions:

1. Combine soaked almonds, banana, shredded coconut, cocoa powder, and almond milk in a blender.
2. Blend until smooth.
3. If desired, add ice cubes and blend again.
4. Pour into a glass and indulge in the almond joyous flavors.

Nutrition Information (per serving):

- Calories: 220
- Protein: 6g
- Carbohydrates: 20g

- Fat: 15g
- Fiber: 6g
- Sugar: 8g
- Portion Size: 1 smoothie

Tropical Turmeric Twist

Ingredients:

- 1 cup pineapple chunks
- 1/2 mango, peeled and sliced
- 1/2 teaspoon turmeric powder
- 1/2 teaspoon ginger, grated
- 1/2 cup plain yogurt
- 1 cup coconut water
- Ice cubes (optional)

Instructions:

1. Combine pineapple, mango, turmeric powder, grated ginger, yogurt, and coconut water in a blender.
2. Blend until smooth.
3. Add ice cubes if desired and blend again.
4. Pour into a glass and enjoy the tropical twist with a hint of turmeric.

Nutrition Information (per serving):

- Calories: 150

- Protein: 5g

- Carbohydrates: 30g

- Fat: 2g

- Fiber: 4g

- Sugar: 20g

- Portion Size: 1 smoothie

Chocolate Avocado Power Smoothie

Ingredients:

- 1/2 avocado

- 1 tablespoon cocoa powder

- 1 banana

- 1 tablespoon honey

- 1 cup almond milk

- Ice cubes (optional)

Instructions:

1. Combine avocado, cocoa powder, banana, honey, and almond milk in a blender.

2. Blend until smooth.

3. If desired, add ice cubes and blend again.

4. Pour into a glass and relish the powerful blend of chocolate and avocado.

Nutrition Information (per serving):

- Calories: 180
- Protein: 4g
- Carbohydrates: 25g
- Fat: 9g
- Fiber: 6g
- Sugar: 15g
- Portion Size: 1 smoothie

Cinnamon Roll Protein Shake

Ingredients:

- 1/2 cup oats
- 1/2 teaspoon cinnamon
- 1 scoop vanilla protein powder
- 1 tablespoon almond butter
- 1 cup milk (dairy or plant-based)
- Ice cubes (optional)

Instructions:

1. Combine oats, cinnamon, protein powder, almond butter, and milk in a blender.
2. Blend until smooth.
3. If desired, add ice cubes and blend again.
4. Pour into a glass and experience the delightful taste of a cinnamon roll in a shake.

Nutrition Information (per serving):

- Calories: 250
- Protein: 20g
- Carbohydrates: 25g
- Fat: 9g
- Fiber: 4g
- Sugar: 8g
- Portion Size: 1 smoothie

Mixed Berry Protein Smoothie

Ingredients:

- 1 cup mixed berries (strawberries, blueberries, raspberries)
- 1 scoop vanilla protein powder

- 1/2 cup Greek yogurt
- 1 tablespoon chia seeds
- 1 cup water
- Ice cubes (optional)

Instructions:

1. Combine mixed berries, protein powder, Greek yogurt, chia seeds, and water in a blender.
2. Blend until smooth.
3. Add ice cubes if desired and blend again.
4. Pour into a glass and relish the protein-packed goodness with a burst of berry flavor.

Nutrition Information (per serving):

- Calories: 160
- Protein: 15g
- Carbohydrates: 20g
- Fat: 3.5g
- Fiber: 6g
- Sugar: 10g
- Portion Size: 1 smoothie

Peachy Green Smoothie

Ingredients:

- 1 cup peaches, sliced
- 1 cup spinach leaves
- 1/2 banana
- 1/2 cup plain yogurt
- 1 tablespoon honey
- 1 cup water
- Ice cubes (optional)

Instructions:

1. Combine peaches, spinach, banana, yogurt, honey, and water in a blender.
2. Blend until smooth.
3. If desired, add ice cubes and blend again.
4. Pour into a glass and savor the delightful combination of peaches and greens.

Nutrition Information (per serving):

- Calories: 130
- Protein: 4g
- Carbohydrates: 25g

- Fat: 2.5g

- Fiber: 4g

- Sugar: 18g

- Portion Size: 1 smoothie

Coffee and Almond Smoothie

Ingredients:

- 1 cup brewed coffee, chilled

- 1/2 banana

- 2 tablespoons almond butter

- 1/2 teaspoon vanilla extract

- 1 cup almond milk

- Ice cubes (optional)

Instructions:

1. Combine chilled coffee, banana, almond butter, vanilla extract, and almond milk in a blender.

2. Blend until smooth.

3. Add ice cubes if desired and blend again.

4. Pour into a glass and enjoy the energizing combination of coffee and almonds.

Nutrition Information (per serving):

- Calories: 180
- Protein: 6g
- Carbohydrates: 15g
- Fat: 12g
- Fiber: 3g
- Sugar: 8g
- Portion Size: 1 smoothie

CONCLUSION

Throughout these chapters, we've navigated the realms of nutritious and delightful culinary experiences, proving that maintaining a diabetes-friendly diet doesn't mean compromising on taste. Each recipe is a testament to the richness of ingredients and the creativity that can be infused into meals while keeping blood sugar levels in check.

The 30-day meal plan serves as a roadmap, guiding you through the intricacies of a balanced and diverse diet. From the energizing breakfasts that kickstart your day to the satisfying dinners that bring it to a close, every dish is a celebration of wholesome goodness.

But this isn't just about meals; it's about fostering a sustainable and enjoyable lifestyle. The snacks and appetizers tantalize the taste buds without jeopardizing your health goals, while the desserts add a touch of sweetness to life without compromising on diabetic considerations.

In the realm of smoothies, we've crafted vibrant concoctions that go beyond mere refreshment – they're liquid vitality, packing nutrition and flavor into every sip.

Remember, this cookbook isn't a set of rules; it's an invitation to explore, experiment, and savor the joys of a diabetes-conscious culinary adventure. It's about finding joy in the kitchen, discovering the versatility of ingredients, and embracing a lifestyle that nourishes both body and soul.

As you embark on this journey, let each recipe be a reminder that managing Type 2 Diabetes is not a restriction but an opportunity to savor a diverse tapestry of flavors. With each mindful bite, you're not just nourishing your body but also sowing the seeds of a vibrant and fulfilling life.

May this cookbook be your trusted guide on a path paved with delicious and healthful choices. Here's to savoring every moment and every bite – to a life well-lived, and well-eaten. Cheers to your health, happiness, and the endless possibilities that lie ahead!